THE LITTLE BOOK OF
BELFAST
SAYINGS

The Little Book of Belfast
Sayings

Steve Holmes

Welcome to the heart of Northern Ireland, where the streets are lined with stories, laughter dances through the air, and the warmth of the people lights up even the rainiest days. "The Little Book of Belfast Sayings" is your personal guide to the soul of this charming city, a place where history and modernity blend seamlessly, creating a culture rich in tradition and vibrant with contemporary life.

Belfast, with its stunning architecture, lush green parks, and bustling markets, is a city that invites exploration and rewards the curious. From the majestic cranes of the Harland and Wolff shipyard, casting their long shadows over the city that built the Titanic, to the peace walls that whisper tales of a complex past, Belfast is a city of contrasts, resilience, and beauty.

But what truly makes Belfast stand out is its people. Belfastians are known for their quick wit, their steadfastness, and their ability to find joy in the everyday. It's a city where a stranger is just a friend you haven't met yet, where every conversation is an opportunity for laughter, and where the local dialect is as rich and flavorful as a pint of the finest stout.

"The Little Book of Belfast Sayings" captures the essence of this splendid city through its unique sayings and phrases. These expressions, collected with love, offer a window into the heart of Belfast's community, showcasing the humor, the warmth, and the unbreakable spirit of its residents. As you turn the pages, you'll be transported to the cobbled streets of Cathedral Quarter, the bustling stalls of St. George's Market, and the tranquil paths of the Botanic Gardens.

This book is not just a collection of sayings; it's an invitation to experience Belfast in its truest form. It's a tribute to the city's beauty, its resilience, and above all, its people. So, whether you're a local looking to nod in agreement and chuckle at the familiar, or a visitor hoping to delve deeper into the Belfast way of life, this book is for you. Let's embark on this journey together, through the heart and soul of Belfast, one saying at a time. Welcome, and enjoy every wee bit of it!

"Grand"

Fine or okay.

"Banjaxed"

Broken or ruined beyond repair.

"Wee buns"

Easy or no problem.

"Dead on"

Perfect, exactly right, or okay.

Belfast Sayings

"Catch yourself on!"

Wise up or stop being
ridiculous.

"What's the craic?"

How are you, or what's happening?

"Bout ye!"

Short for "How about you?" A common greeting.

"Scundered"

Embarrassed or ashamed.

"Wind your neck in"

Mind your own business or
stop being nosy.

"Your guddies are scrappers"

Your shoes are bad. No good.

"You're a geg"

You're funny or
entertaining.

"Pure beaut"

Really beautiful or
excellent.

"Wile"

Very or terrible, depending on context. "Wile good" or "Wile weather."

"Our kid"

A term of endearment for a younger sibling or close friend.

"Keep 'er lit"

Keep going or maintain
your current course of
action.

"Ragin"

Very angry.

"Suckin' diesel"

Now we're making
progress or succeeding.

"The back of beyond"

A place that's far away or remote.

"It's Baltic"

It's very cold.

"Aye"

Yes.

"Guddies"

Sneakers or casual shoes.

"Right enough"

Indeed, or you're correct.

"Give my head peace"

Leave me alone or stop annoying me.

"Stickin' out"

Great or fantastic.

"Deadly"

Really good or impressive.

"Does my head in"

Annoys or frustrates me.

"Cracker"

Excellent or very good.

"Norn Iron"

Phonetically how some locals say "Northern Ireland".

"Sound"

Reliable or trustworthy;
also used to mean okay.

"Go 'way on"

Expression of disbelief or amazement. Or tell someone to move out of your sight.

"Here's me wha?"

Used when telling a story
to introduce direct speech
or thought.

"Faffin'"

Wasting time or dilly-dallying.

"Keks"

Trousers or pants.

"Yarn"

A story, often an exaggerated one.

"Knackered"

Very tired or exhausted.

"Melter"

Someone or something
that is intensely annoying
or frustrating.

"Peelers"

Police, derived from Sir
Robert Peel, founder of
the modern police force.

"Quare"

An intensifier, meaning very or extremely. "Quare good."

"Tea"

Dinner or the evening meal.

"Fein"

Man or person, sometimes
used in a derogatory sense.

"Jammy"

Lucky or fortuitous.

"Buck eejit"

A term of endearment for
someone acting foolishly.

"Dander"

A leisurely walk. "Going for a dander."

"Full whack"

At full price or maximum speed.

"Gobsmacked"

Astonished or amazed.

"Hoak"

To search or rummage
through something.

"Lethal"

Really cool or awesome.

"Manky"

Dirty, disgusting, or
unpleasant.

"Natter"

A long and casual
conversation.

"Oul"

A prefix meaning old but
used affectionately.

"Poke"

Ice cream cone.

"Quid"

Slang for pounds sterling.

"Reddener"

A blush or feeling of
embarrassment.

"Sesh"

A period of time spent
engaging in an activity,
usually drinking.

"Tayto sandwich"

A sandwich made with crisps, named after the popular brand.

"Up to high doh"

Extremely anxious or
excited.

"Vexed"

Annoyed, frustrated, or angry.

"Wrecked"

Extremely tired or
destroyed.

"Yoke"

Thing or object often used when the speaker can't remember the specific name.

"Zonked"

Completely exhausted.

"Belter"

Something considered
excellent or amazing.

"I'm Off to the Devinish"

Going to see an adult night out drinking.

"Culchie"

A country person or person
not from the city.

"Violumpet man"

A famous street performer
many knew in Belfast.

"Yeoo"

Expression of happiness
and proudness.

"Yousins"

Everyone as a group.

"You owe me a tenner"

You are in debt to a person
In the amount of 10 pound
coins.

"Up the 'mona bypass"

Great respects to this area of Belfast.

"Yous' love your mcdonalds, don't ye"

Stating to people that they enjoy eating food.

"That's so north down"

That is very posh of you to say or do.

"You wouldn't be long getting frostbit"

It is very cold.

"Half on"

Not fully committed or
only somewhat interested.

"Like a bull in a China shop"

Behaving recklessly or clumsily in a situation that requires care.

"On the tear"

Going out with the intention of drinking or partying.

"Pure dead brilliant"

Absolutely fantastic or excellent.

"Rattled"

Upset, disturbed, or very annoyed.

"She's a dote"

She's very sweet,
endearing, or adorable.

"The dogs on the street know"

Common knowledge or very obvious.

"Thon"

That or those, often used
to specify something at a
distance.

"Under the weather"

Feeling ill or not oneself.

"Wheesht"

Be quiet or hush.

"Your head's a
Marley"

You're not thinking
straight or talking
nonsense.

"A face as long as a Lurgan spade"

Looking very unhappy or discontented.

"Buckled"

Laughing uncontrollably.

"Donkey's years"

A very long time.

"Falling from the heavens"

Raining very heavily.

"Give it a lash"

To try something or give it
a go.

"Happy out"

Content or satisfied with
the situation.

"Not worth a button"

Of no value or importance.

"Away on with ye"

Disbelief at what someone is saying or telling them to stop exaggerating.

"He's not worth his salt"

He's not worth what he's paid or not very good at what he does.

"Like a headless chicken"

Acting in a frantic or disorganized manner.

"Mad as a box of frogs"

Very crazy or eccentric.

"Not a bother"

No problem or easily done.

"Over the moon"

Extremely happy or
pleased.

"Speak of the devil"

The person we were just talking about has appeared.

"The bee's knees"

Something that is of excellent or very high quality.

"The full Monty"

Everything that is
available or possible.

"Thrown under the bus"

Betrayed or sacrificed for the benefit of others.

"Tight as a duck's arse"

Very stingy or not generous.

"Two sandwiches short of a picnic"

Not very intelligent or a bit mad.

"Up to ninety"

Very busy or agitated.

"Wouldn't pull the wool over her eyes"

Can't deceive her easily.

"You can't make a silk purse out of a sow's ear"

You can't create something good from something bad.

"Your eyes are bigger than your belly"

You've taken more food than you can eat.

"A watched pot never boils"

Time feels slower when you're waiting for something to happen.

"Barking up the wrong tree"

Looking in the wrong place or accusing the wrong person.

"Having a giraffe"

Having a laugh or joking about.

As we wrap up our journey through the linguistic landscape of Belfast and Northern Ireland, it's clear that the local vernacular is much more than just a way of speaking. It's a reflection of the city's history, its culture, and most importantly, its people. The sayings we've explored, from the humorous to the poignant, offer a glimpse into the everyday lives of those who call this vibrant city home. They reveal a community rich in storytelling, marked by resilience, and imbued with a unique sense of humour that can find light even in the darkest of times.

"The Little Book of Belfast Sayings" is not merely a collection of phrases; it's an invitation to experience the heart and soul of Belfast. Each saying, each expression, is a thread in the larger tapestry of Northern Irish culture, woven together by generations of shared experiences. As you close the pages of this book, it's our hope that you carry with you a piece of Belfast, a reminder of the warmth, wit, and wisdom that define this remarkable city.

Whether you're a local reminiscing on familiar phrases, an expatriate feeling a tug at your heartstrings, or a visitor enchanted by the city's charm, these sayings serve as a bridge connecting us all. They remind us that, no matter where we go, the spirit of Belfast and the warmth of its people are never far behind.

So, here's to Belfast — a city of history, of beauty, and of laughter. May its sayings continue to inspire, amuse, and bring us together, no matter where we find ourselves in the world.

Thank you for exploring "The Little Book of Belfast Sayings" with us. If you've enjoyed the journey, we kindly invite you to share your experience by leaving a five-star review on Amazon. Your support helps us reach more readers and celebrate the rich linguistic heritage of Belfast together.

Printed in Great Britain
by Amazon